LIFE IN EXTREME ENVIRONMENTS™

LIFE AT A HIGH ALTITUDE

JUDY LEVIN

rosen
central™

The Rosen Publishing Group, Inc., New York

For Laura

Published in 2004 by The Rosen Publishing Group, Inc.
29 East 21st Street, New York, NY 10010

Library of Congress Cataloging-in-Publication Data

Levin, Judy, 1956–
Life at a high altitude/Judy Levin.—1st ed.
   p. cm.—(Life in extreme environments)
Summary: Defines high altitudes, where air is thinner, cooler, and drier, and indicates how plants, animals, and humans learn to survive in this extreme environment.
Includes bibliographical references.
ISBN 0-8239-3987-1 (lib. bdg.)
1. Altitude, Influence of—Juvenile literature. [1. Altitude, Influence of. 2. Mountains. 3. Mountain ecology. 4. Ecology. 5. Survival.]
I. Title. II. Series.
QP82.2.A4L48 2004
577.5'3–dc21
                                    2003002182

Manufactured in the United States of America

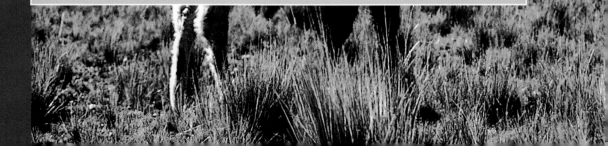

CONTENTS

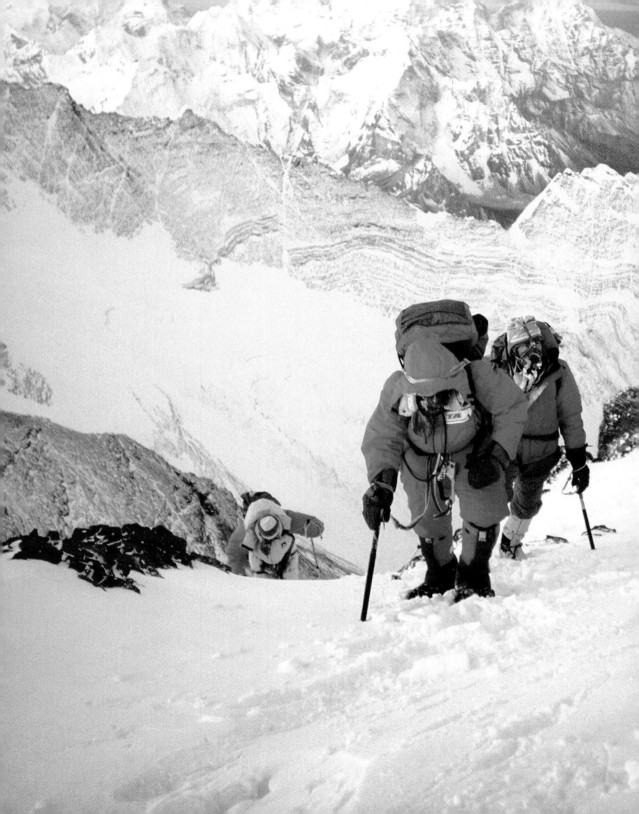

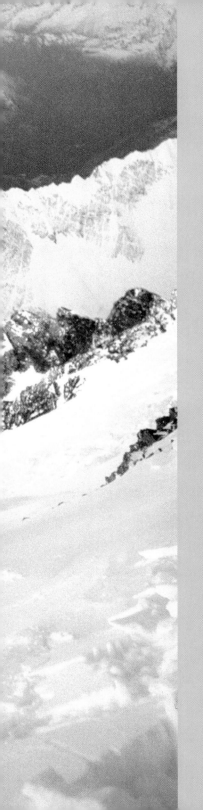

INTRODUCTION: THIN AIR

Almost 2,000 years ago, a Chinese general who marched his army through high mountains named them Mount Greater Headache, Mount Lesser Headache, and Fever Hill. Even the horses on the journey got sick. Travelers reported dragons in the mountains as late as the 1700s. Later, they didn't find dragons, but people realized that something odd happened at high altitudes. They got headaches. They also felt tired, cold, dizzy, and dried out. And they couldn't sleep. Some people threw up and others died. Maybe the strange plants and minerals were poisonous, they thought. But no one really knew what was happening.

Then, in 1787, a Swiss mountaineer named Horace Benedict de Saussure

Hikers climbing Mount Everest in Nepal. Despite modern technology that helps climbers keep warm and breathe freely at high altitudes, many people are still injured or killed climbing Everest, the world's tallest mountain.

took a barometer to the top of France's Mont Blanc—15,771 feet (4,802 meters)—and measured the weight of the air. The barometer showed that the atmosphere was lighter on top of Mont Blanc than at sea level. He had discovered thin air.

Usually, we take air for granted. But it's there, made of molecules rushing around and bumping into one another. Earth's atmosphere is heaviest at the bottom and then thins out little by little until there's nothing left but space. At 29,028 feet (8,848 m) on top of Mount Everest in the Himalayas, air is a quarter of its sea-level weight. At the summit of Everest, you can't take the atmosphere for granted. You're 5.5 miles up (almost 9 kilometers) and you're running out of air.

At about 8,000 feet (2,400 m) above sea level, most people and some animals have trouble breathing. But even at less extreme altitudes, thin air changes the environment. There are fewer molecules, so they create less heat. Thin air holds less heat so that even on a very hot day a mountain becomes cold at night. And thin air lets the sun's ultraviolet rays through—the rays that cause sunburn and skin cancer. High on a mountain, you can get frostbite and sunburn the same day. Also, changing temperatures and air density can create hurricane-strength winds. As warm air rises and cools, it holds less water vapor, so the air releases rain or snow. The air then becomes cooler and drier, dehydrating every plant, animal, and person around.

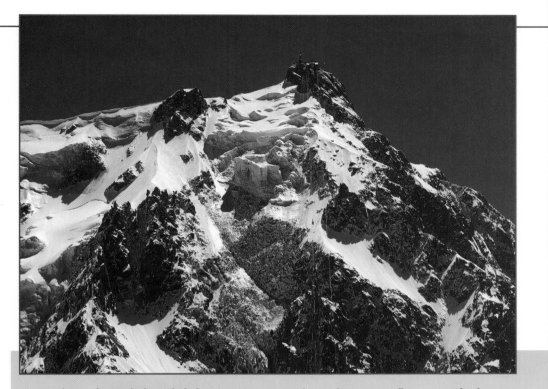

Mont Blanc, in the French Alps, is the highest mountain in Europe. The French sometimes call it *La Dame Blanche*, "The White Lady." It is popular with climbers and skiers from all over Europe.

Regardless of these extremes, thousands of species of plants and animals live at high altitudes. In 2001, about 140 million people lived at 8,000 feet (2,400 m) or higher. How is it that they are able to survive? They have adapted.

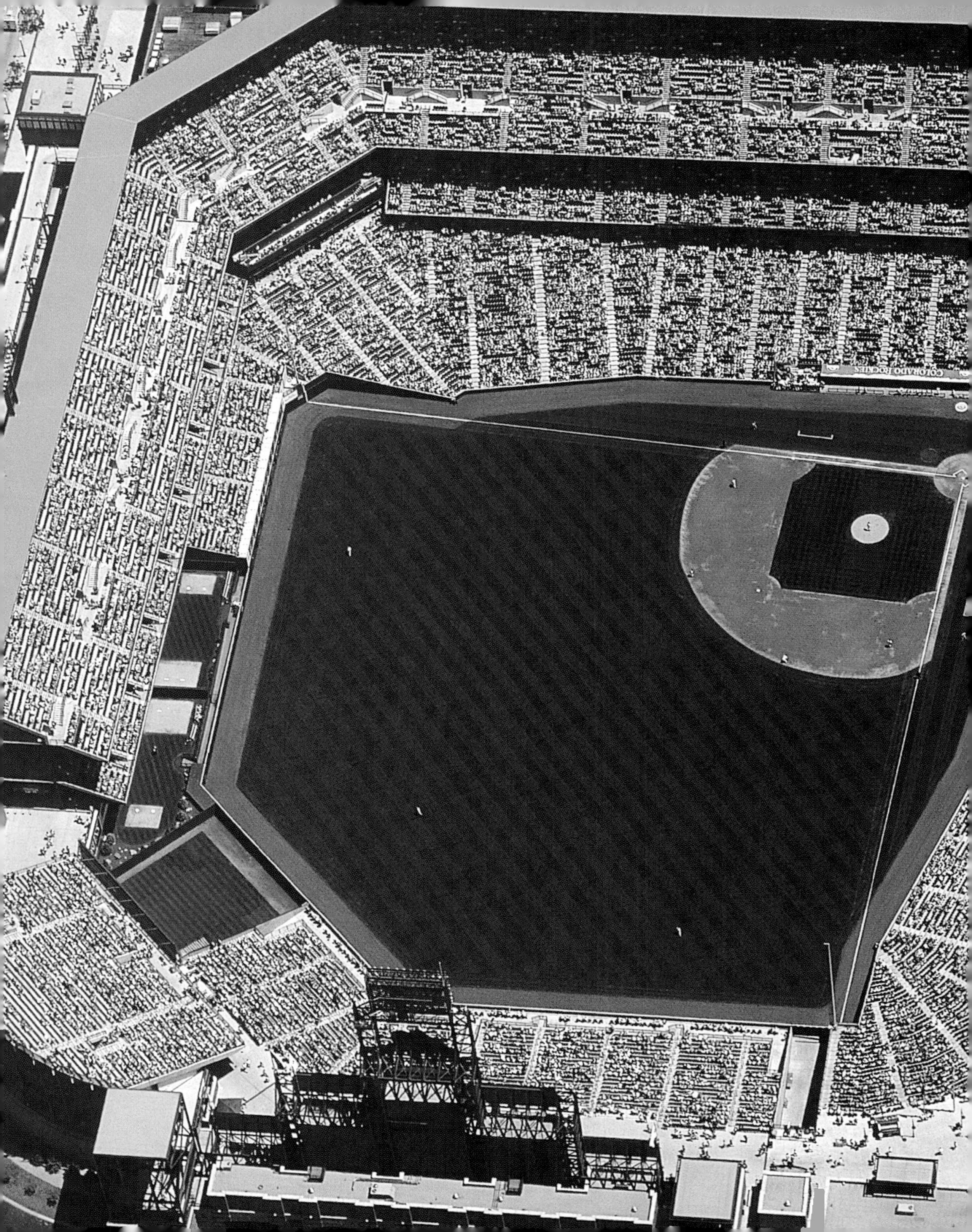
COLORADO ROCKIES

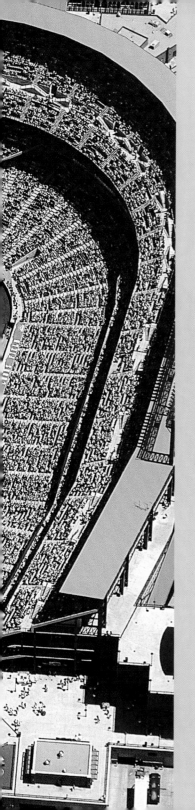

CHAPTER ONE

HANGING ON FOR THEIR LIVES

A baseball can't adapt to high altitudes. At Coors Field in Denver, players hit a lot of home runs. At one mile up (1,609 m), thin air allows a baseball to soar. Pitchers complained that the baseballs felt funny, and they were right. Because mountain air dries out baseballs, they weigh less than at sea level. Coors Field baseballs are now stored in big humidors—containers originally designed to keep cigars fresh—because they make the air more humid.

Baseballs can't adapt to high altitudes, but plants can. Of course, that doesn't mean any plant can grow at any altitude. A plant doesn't need much oxygen, but it is affected by thin air in other ways.

LOTS OF SNOW, NOT MUCH SOIL

Suppose you want to plant a maple tree 15,000 feet (4,500 m) above sea level. However, high on a mountain slope, soil blows and washes away faster than it can form. If you plant your maple in a large pot of soil that you have somehow dragged up the mountain, your maple still can't grow. Its thin flat leaves shrivel in the dry air. Snow falling on its leafy branches snaps them off. The daytime sun makes the maple's sap flow. The icy nighttime temperatures make the sap freeze. You hear a noise like a shot: it's the sound of a maple tree exploding as the frozen sap suddenly expands. Deciduous trees—trees with flat leaves that change color and fall off— are not adapted to high altitudes.

What kind of plants can grow on a mountain? It depends on where the mountain is and where the plant is on the mountain. A 3,000-foot (900-m) mountain in Antarctica is ice and rock, but 9,000 feet (2,750 m) up Mount Kenya

Mount Kenya, the second-highest mountain in Africa, is on the equator yet has a peak covered in snow. It is located in the Central Highlands area, where the soil is fertile enough to grow wheat. Mount Kenya National Park is on the upper slopes of the mountain.

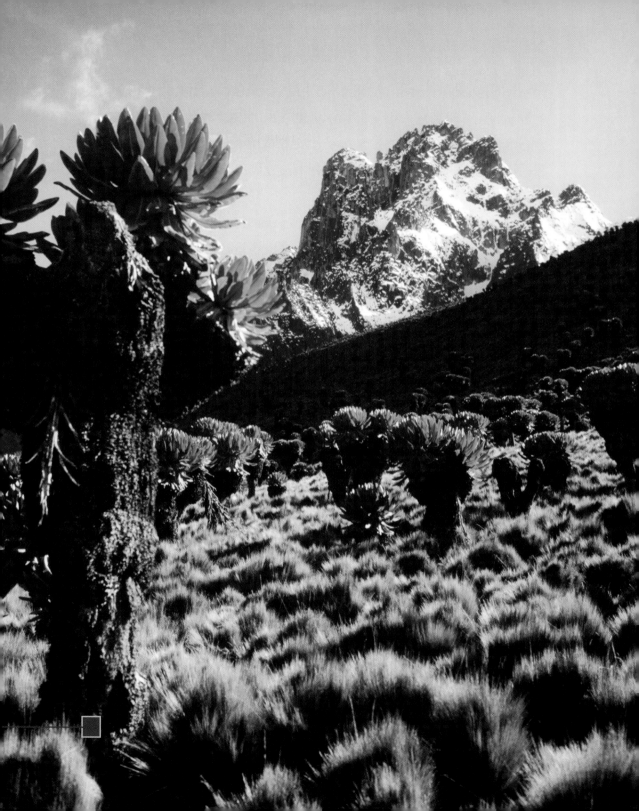

(near the equator in Africa) a lush bamboo forest grows. However, at the top of the world's tallest mountains, plants are not able to grow at all. There is no soil, every night the temperature is below freezing, and the howling winds create blizzards.

High up any tall mountain is a permanent snow line. Above it, there is snow all year. That line is the limit of where plants can grow, except in tiny protected patches. As you go farther down, the mountain comes to life. It may still look as though it's all ice and rock, but patches of color appear. Red algae, lichens, mosses—these are able to survive extreme conditions. They barely look like plants, but they're alive and growing (though quite slowly). Lichens can get nourishment directly from the rock, and they might grow one quarter of an inch (less than 0.5 centimeter) in hundreds of years.

The ability to grow slowly and to wait out the coldest times is shared by all extreme altitude plants. When you're cold, you wrap your arms around yourself and curl up in a ball to conserve heat. If you're in a high wind, you hunker down so the wind won't knock you over, or you find a little niche where rocks protect you—even a hole in the ground. Many animals and plants living at extreme altitudes do the same thing.

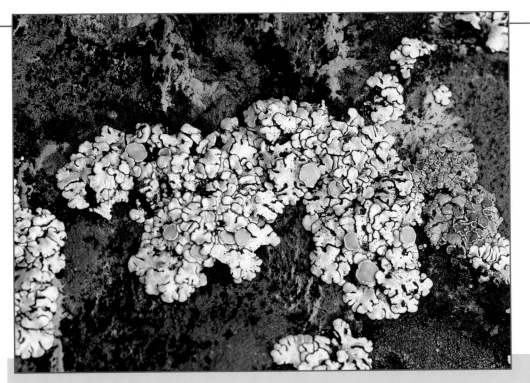

Lichens are among the toughest and most widespread life forms on Earth. They can even be found on rocks in the Antarctic. Estimates of known species vary from 13,500 to 17,000, but since only an estimated 50-70 percent of them are known, there may be as many as 20,000 species in all. Temperate rain forests have the greatest diversity of lichens, but lichens make up most of the plant life in Arctic and Alpine habitats.

Tough Plants

Soil is composed of ground-up rock, water, and decayed plants and animals. Up a mountain, soil is scarcely there at all. It washes away, it blows away, and it has trouble forming in the first place. Up near the level of permanent snow, plants have to find tiny pockets of soil that have collected between rocks. Naturalists sometimes call them "belly plants" because you have to lie on your stomach to study them.

Some, like snow buttercups, grow under the snow, using it as a fluffy blanket and basking in the sun whenever possible. Other belly plants, such as edelweiss, grow hair or even fur that provides warmth and helps keep the plant from drying out. Other plants make antifreeze, adding oils to the water

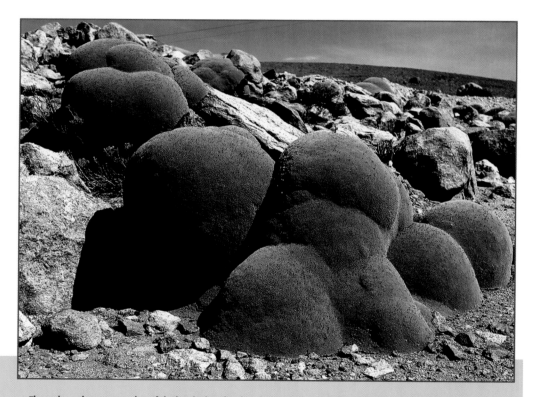

The cushion plant is a member of the heath plant family, which includes cranberries, blueberries, and rhododendrons. Like moss, cushion plants have large root systems that allow them to attach to rocky landscapes.

they've stored in their leaves. This keeps their food supply drinkable even when the temperature drops below freezing.

The other plants that do well up near the snow line are "cushion plants." These are fat, dense, and round. Most are not a single plant, but whole colonies of plants that huddle together for warmth and protection. The wind goes over the cushion instead of through it, so the center of the plant stays warm and wet. Like the belly plants, they grow very bright flowers, and the vibrant colors attract insects, which then fertilize them. Other plants actually heat up and melt the snow around them.

All of these plants send their roots deep into the ground, hanging on tight against the winds and sucking up every bit of food and water they can. A 2-inch-tall (5-cm) plant may send its roots 12 inches (30.5 cm) down or wrap them around a rock like a net. A few plants are so tough that only the largest avalanche will uproot them.

Plants with Fur

Near the permanent snow line, plants are similar all over the world. As you move lower down, there is more variation. Mountains in Europe and the United States have alpine meadows, named for the European Alps, where there are fields of flowering deep-rooted plants. Yet in a tropical alpine

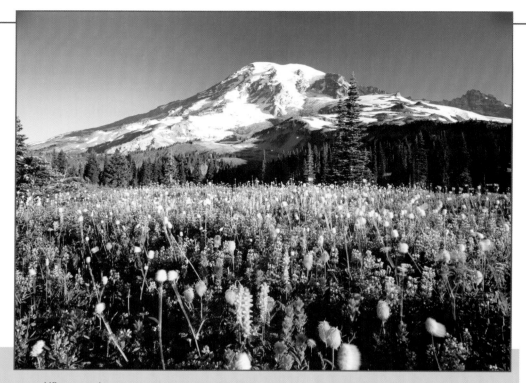

A wildflower meadow near Mount Rainier in Washington State. The mountain is actually an active volcano encased in over 35 square miles (about 90 sq km) of snow and ice. As many as 10,000 climbers attempt to reach its summit every year. Due to rapid weather changes and altitude gain, only about half of those who attempt to reach the top actually make it.

field, giant lobelias grow—shaggy, silver-furred plants that can grow to be as tall as an adult human. Like the small alpine plants, they are protected from the harsh sun and cold nights by their fur, but in the Tropics, they do not have long winters to slow down their growth.

Lower still on a mountain, the depth of the snow controls the height of some plants. A small tree will put out new growth in the summer. When winter comes, any part of that tree that isn't under the snow gets torn off by the wind. As the trees age, they twist and grow crooked, but they can't grow taller. Then, finally, you come to the timberline: the altitude below which trees can live and grow normally. On some mountains, you will never come to this line. Near the Arctic and the Antarctic, the weather is too cold for trees. These are Earth's timberlines, where summer temperatures stay below 50° Fahrenheit (10° Celsius).

But even at the timberline, you can't plant a maple. The trees that can survive at the highest altitude are the conifers—evergreen trees that produce cones. The sticky resin in their needles is an antifreeze. Their skinny needles don't lose heat and moisture as fast as flat leaves. The conifers' flexible branches can blow in the wind without snapping. In a heavy snowfall, a conifer's branches bow down under the snow's weight, like an umbrella folding up. Conifers can also grow year-round. If there's warmth, they grow. If it's cold, they wait.

By the time you reach the mountain height that can support a conifer, you're not in extreme altitudes anymore. What grows there? Rain forest? Desert? A forest of maple and other deciduous trees? It all depends on what mountain you just came down.

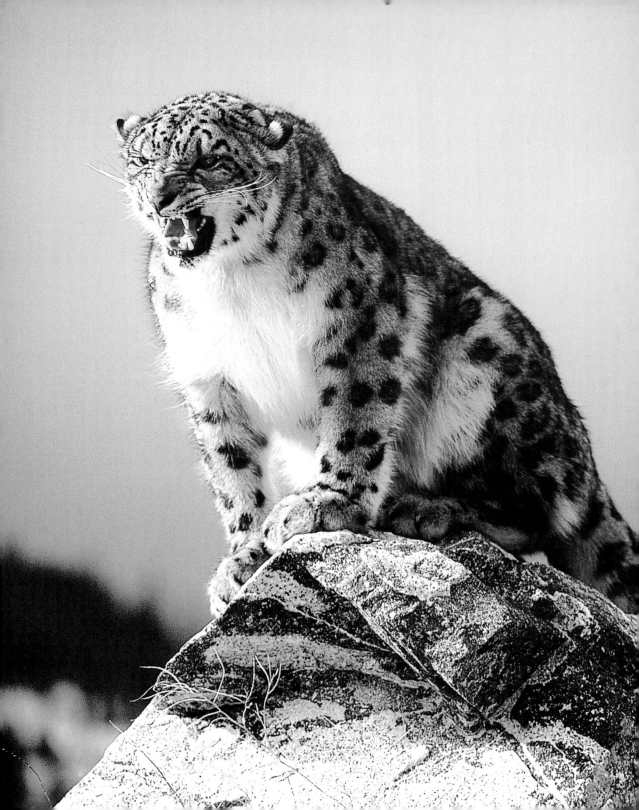

CHAPTER TWO
SURVIVORS OF THE ANIMAL WORLD

Plants can ignore the lack of oxygen at extreme altitudes, but animals can't. Because they don't have roots, they have to make sure that they don't blow off the mountain. They also must cope with extreme temperature variations.

On top of Aconcagua (22,834 feet/6,969 m), the tallest mountain in South America's Andes, you are not expecting company. No animals live there. But look up. Is that a plane? No, it's a vulture—or the Andean condor. The largest

A snow leopard crouches on a rock. Snow leopards are generally found in the Middle East and Asia, including Afghanistan, China, India, and Russia. They have large, well-cushioned paws, a strong chest, and short forelimbs that enable them to scale high cliffs. Snow leopards will prey on wild sheep and goats, but they also eat marmots, pikas, hares, and game birds, as well as domestic sheep and goats—which can make them targets for local hunters.

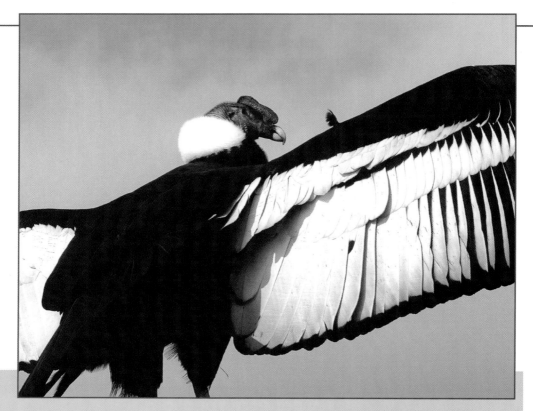

The Andean condor, like its relative, the Californian condor, is a carrion feeder who will sometimes attack small or wounded prey. Andean condor chicks take about two years to raise. Once raised, condors do not mate until they are eight to ten years old. The fluffy feathers on the condor's neck are a cold weather adaptation; when it moves certain muscles, the feathers will rise and cover the back of its head.

wingspan of any bird in the world—about 10 feet (3.5 m)—helps keep the 28-pound (12.6-kilogram) condor airborne, and like all vultures, it has a taste for dead meat. Animals that don't survive the extreme climate become vulture lunch. The vultures really can look like planes: they don't flap their wings—they soar.

High Fliers and Small Floaters

Because of the thin air, an airplane needs an extra-long runway to take off from El Alto, the airport on Bolivia's high plains, but the Andean condor takes off quite comfortably, unless it has a full stomach. Birds have great respiratory systems, meant to let them use a lot of energy high up. Geese migrate at higher altitudes than Mount Everest, protected by the same stuff that protects you when you put on a down-filled jacket. Down is the soft feathers near the bird's skin.

Other inhabitants of the roof of the world are even more unexpected: insects and spiders. They do not walk or fly to 22,000 feet (6,700 m) but float upward—blown up the mountain by air currents. Those same upward drafts bring them daily food deliveries of pollen, seeds, and dead insects. Why don't they freeze? Because like many lowland insects, they become dormant in the extreme cold. They look dead, but when the sun warms them, they wake up again. Many of them are darker than their lowland relatives, so they absorb heat more easily. Their dark colors also protect them from harmful ultraviolet rays. Insects don't have lungs. They breathe through tubes that lead from their exterior skeleton. Thin air doesn't bother them.

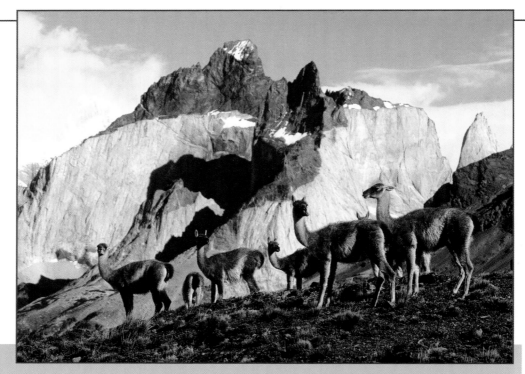

Guanacos, above, can be found all over South and Central America, from the tip of Tierra del Fuego to the Andes. They are somewhat smaller than llamas but are otherwise very similar. Guanacos are wild and endangered in much of their range, although attempts are now being made to protect them, especially in Argentina.

Shaggy Mountaineers

Llamas (in the Andes) and yaks (in the Himalayas) have been domesticated for thousands of years, and the people of those regions could not survive without them. They live at the highest altitudes of any large mammals. Llamas and their relatives— vicuñas, guanacos, and alpacas—have dense shaggy fur coats to keep them warm and to help repel rain. The ability to survive the cold is an important adaptation high in the Andes.

The wild guanaco's coat is different thicknesses on different parts of its body. It can't quite unzip its coat, but almost. On a hot day, the thinner fur on its stomach keeps it from overheating. When it's cold, the animal curls up, so that the thicker fur on its back and neck covers all of it.

Llamas, vicuñas, guanacos, and alpacas are related to each other—and to the camel. Like camels everywhere, they're adapted to dry conditions. They can chew and digest tough, thorny plants that most animals couldn't eat. They don't urinate much. The guanaco doesn't need to drink at all. It gets enough water from the plants it eats. But these highland "camels" have narrow feet with two separate toes —while the desert camel's toes are webbed. The guanaco's toes help it keep its balance on rocky paths and steep cliffs.

Llamas and their relatives also have adaptations that cannot be seen: high red blood cell counts. Red blood cells collect oxygen from the lungs and carry it to every part of the body. Extra red blood cells give the llama more oxygen, enough to live in very thin air. Other animals can adapt to high altitudes by developing more red blood cells, but the llama doesn't need to; it has them all the time. Llamas are fairly good-looking—vicuñas are even elegant—but elegance is not an adaptation to extreme altitudes. That is a lucky thing for the yak, which is not elegant at all.

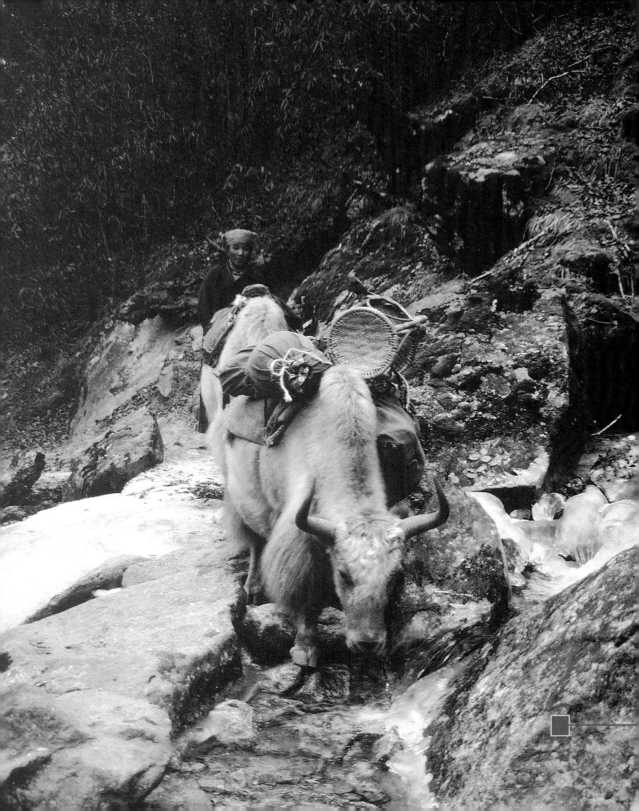

The Yak

A very large hairy ox, the yak is comfortable above 20,000 feet (6,100 m), higher than any other large mammal. Everything you see on a yak is an adaptation. Its dark shaggy body conserves heat and energy, as do its neck, short legs, and tail. As with high-altitude plants, "fat" and "hairy" are qualities that protect high-altitude animals. Yaks do not get sunburned. And because they stay warm, they do not burn extra calories. Since a yak has a light diet—grass—it doesn't have a lot of extra calories to burn.

The yak's short legs are strong. Its hooves are small and sharp. When the yak is hauling its 880-pound (396-kg) self down a steep mountain, it has to be careful not to slip, trip, or slide. Its sharp hooves dig into the ground and keep it from slipping to its death. The yak's boxy shape allows for a big heart and big lungs. Yaks breathe deeply and often. Like the llamas, they have extra red blood cells. Additionally, each of these blood cells holds more oxygen than a lowland cow's red blood cells. Thus, a yak is able to breathe in very thin air.

The yak was probably domesticated in Tibet during the first millennium BC and is now found throughout the high plateaus and mountains of central Asia. Yaks found in zoos are usually of the domesticated variety, which is smaller than the wild yak. There are now more than 12 million domestic yaks (such as the one at left) in the highlands of central Asia.

Small, Fat, and Furry

Heat loss is a problem for small animals. A chinchilla will suffer from the cold more than a llama. In the same way that its long tail is a chill risk, it has a lot more outside surface area in relation to its inside area. The many small

OTHER FAMOUS ADAPTATIONS

- **The Himalayan snow leopard has a fat furry tail for warmth and fur on the bottoms of its extra-wide paws so it won't slip.**

- **Mountain goats and sheep have great balance and built-in shock absorbers: they can step off a cliff while grazing and land, still chewing, 20 feet (6 m) down, on footholds too small for us to see.**

- **The snowshoe hare really does have paws like snowshoes that allow it to hop on the surface of the snow without falling through.**

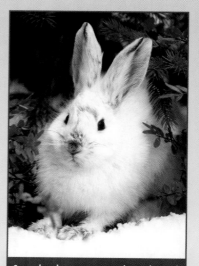

Snowshoe hares are very shy and spend most of the day hiding in shallow depressions, venturing out to eat at night, dusk, and early morning.

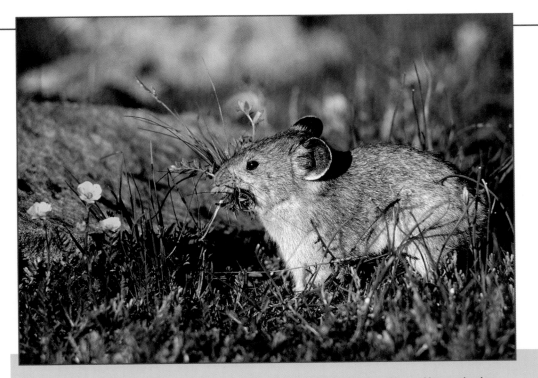

The pika, also called a mouse hare or rock rabbit, is a short-haired mammal related to rabbits and hares. Pikas live above the timberline in the mountains of northern Asia and western North America. The pika differs from the rabbit in that its body is smaller and the ears on its blunt head are shorter; also unlike the rabbit, the front and back legs of a pika are about equal in length. Because food is difficult to obtain in winter in the harsh tundra environment, pikas cut, sun-dry, and store vegetation to use in the winter.

animals that live high in the mountains of the world—pikas, chinchillas, marmots, guinea pigs, snowshoe hares, hyrax, and others—look somewhat alike, even though they are different species.

These small mammals are almost all compact and furry. Even the skinny ones curl up for warmth. Hares in the desert have huge flat ears to cool them down, but hares who live at high altitudes have shorter ears. Tails are often short, but if they are long, they are furry and can be wrapped around the animal like a scarf.

These small animals still need other adaptations for the coldest parts of the year. Some of them can conduct their winter lives in tunnels under the snow. Most of them burrow deep into the ground. These underground tunnels (like their snow tunnels) help them stay warm and escape their enemies. This is also where they raise their young.

Some of these little vegetarians, like the marmot, hibernate in the winter. The snowshoe hare does not, but it turns from brown to white, so predators cannot see it against the snow. The pika has a more unusual adaptation. It mows down plants with its big front teeth, dries them in the sun, and then stores them under rocks. This, however, is a sparse diet, so the pika also eats its own nighttime droppings.

WHEN IS AN ADAPTATION NOT AN ADAPTATION?

Andean wild chinchillas were nearly hunted to extinction because their beautiful fluffy coats were sought after by manufacturers of fur coats. Although chinchillas are now farm-raised for their fur and the wild ones have been allowed to multiply in peace, what started as a great cold-weather adaptation turned into a problem. Other animals have been less lucky. Many species, including the Himalayan snow leopard, will probably disappear forever, killed off for their beautiful fur.

Daytime droppings are too dry, but the nighttime ones have a layer of slime that grows a vitamin-rich layer in the morning sun. It seems like a gross way to get vitamins, but it works for the pikas.

Cold Blood, Warm Skin

One of the first things you learn about animals is that reptiles are cold-blooded—their body temperature is the temperature of their environment. At 16,000 feet (4,900 m), most reptiles would freeze. Yet some high-altitude iguanas wake up with a body temperature of only 35°F (1.5°C). In the cold, their bodies turn a darker color. Then they crawl slowly to a small rock or tuft of grass and expose their whole bodies to the sun. Even on a very cold day, the lizards warm right up.

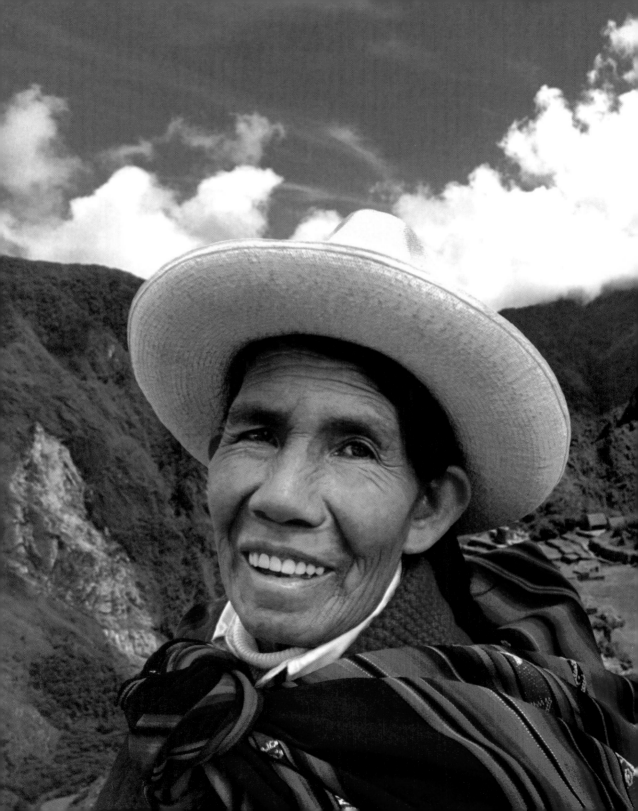

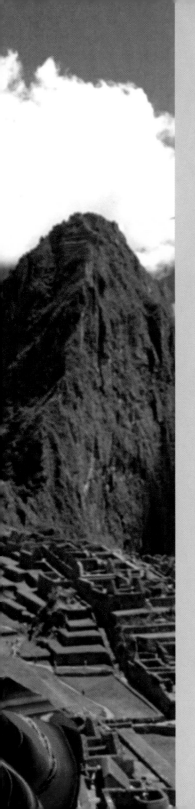

CHAPTER THREE

THE HIGH LIFE

Human beings living at high altitudes have had to adapt, too. Some of these adaptations are not surprising. If the weather is cold and the sun's rays are strong, people put on coats and hats. People who live above the timberline build warm houses of adobe (mud brick) or stone. People are proud of their ability to change the environment to fit their needs. However, humans are not able to make the air hold more oxygen.

Most healthy lowlanders (people who live near sea level) can adapt to lower oxygen within about six

A Quechuan woman standing near Machu Picchu. The Quechua are descendants of the ancient Inca people who, by the 1500s, ruled much of western South America. Numbering about 12 million, they live in Ecuador, Peru, Chile, Argentina, Paraguay, Brazil, and Bolivia. About 2.2 million live in rural areas and speak only Quechua.

weeks. The process of adapting is called acclimatization. This is when the body makes more red blood cells. People find that they can breathe comfortably at 12,000 feet (3,650 m) or more, though they still tire more easily than at sea level. But people who have lived for thousands of years at extreme altitudes have adapted more completely than lowlanders. Some of the adaptations are cultural: over time, people learn how to live in a harsh environment. Other adaptations are biological: like other living things, people have evolved.

THE HIGH PLAINS

Two tribes of indigenous people live in the Andes mountains in South America—the Aymara and the Quechua. Some live on a huge plateau between the northern and southern Andes, a 400,000-square-mile (1,040,000-square-km) area called the Altiplano ("high plain"), which is an average of 12,000 to 14,000 feet (3,650 to 4,250 m) above sea level. There are modern cities in the Altiplano, inhabited by both indigenous peoples and those of European descent. Some Aymara and Quechua live higher up in the mountains.

Their cultural adaptations are the things they have learned over the 6,000 years they have lived in the mountains. Only certain crops will grow high up, such as quinoa (pronounced KEEN-wah) and more than a thousand kinds

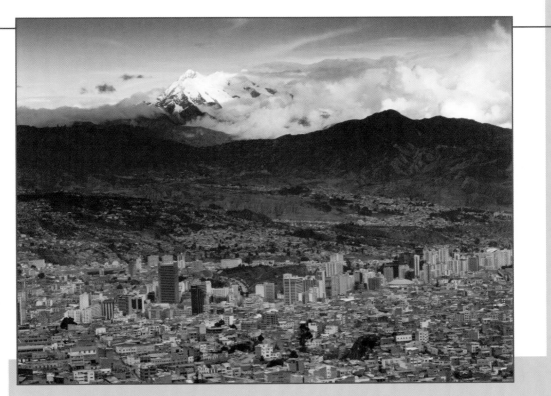

The city of La Paz, the capital of Bolivia. Bolivia has been called the Tibet of the Americas, since it is the highest and most isolated of the Latin American countries. More than 50 percent of the population still maintain their traditional values, beliefs, and ways of life.

of potatoes. Like mountain people everywhere, the Andeans build terraces, which create narrow walled fields for planting food; otherwise, the crops would wash to the bottom of the mountain. Years before modern food companies reinvented the process, Andeans freeze-dried their potatoes for storage, pounding the moisture out of them and drying them in the sun. They brought pieces of glacier down the mountains to cool their food.

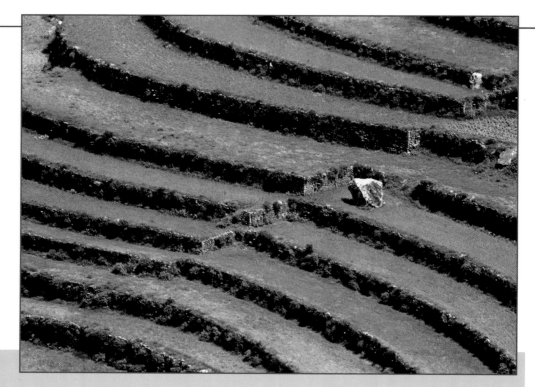

Archaeologists excavate the ancient Incan terraces of Peru. Due to the steep sides of the Incan valleys, terracing and irrigation were vital agricultural techniques. Most of the Incan terraces and canals have been in ruins since the Spanish conquest and are only now being reconstructed.

They salted and dried llama meat and made it into charqui (pronounced CHAR-kee)—from which we get the word "jerky," though North Americans eat dried beef. The Andeans learned that the human body burns more calories in thin air. In hard times, children would go up the mountains to graze the llamas, because a small person needs fewer calories to do the work than a big one.

None of these adaptations make the air less thin. Even on the Altiplano, the air is so thin that cars need specially adapted motors to run. How have the Andean people adapted to extreme altitudes? Like many high-altitude mammals, the Andean Indians have more red blood cells in their blood than lowlanders, even acclimatized lowlanders. They also have more blood in their bodies and larger hearts and lungs to collect oxygen and pump it around. They have slightly shorter arms and legs and

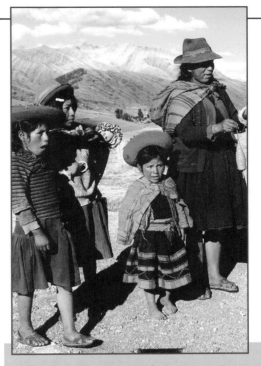

A family of Quechans in Peru. Family ties are very strong among Quechan tribes and extend to complex relationships between neighbors, relatives, and godparents.

more capillaries (small blood vessels) in their hands and feet, protecting their hands and feet from frostbite by bringing more blood to them. (You can warm your feet by stamping them because that brings the blood rushing to the capillaries. Extra capillaries mean the Andeans can bear more cold before they need to start stamping.) The indigenous Andeans have somewhat darker skin than Europeans living in the Altiplano. The dark pigment helps protect them from ultraviolet rays and it helps prevent skin cancer. Andean Indians can suffer from all the altitude problems that lowlanders do, but they will usually develop these problems at a much higher altitude than a lowlander would.

THE HIGHEST LIFE OF ALL

The people who live on the Plateau of Tibet north of Mount Everest and the Sherpas of Nepal on its south, live at the most extreme altitude of anyone in the world. The Plateau of Tibet is 800,000 square miles (2,080,000 square km)—about the size of New York State—and between 13,000 and 15,000 feet (3,700 and 4,575 m) above sea level.

By the early 1900s, mountain climbing had become a popular sport, and Europeans began getting lost in the Himalayas. They couldn't even find the bottoms of the mountains. English explorers hired Sherpas to guide them and to carry equipment, and eventually, Sherpas developed a reputation for being excellent porters. Even now, many mountain climbers use the term Sherpa to mean "porter" or "native guide." But Sherpa is the name of a tribe, not a job description.

Like the Andeans, the Sherpas and other Tibetans (who have been around for about 50,000 years) are well adapted to high altitudes. Tibetans build stone houses and terrace the land for planting food. Instead of llamas they have yaks, which are even more useful than llamas. Yaks will pull a plow and will not spit at you. They provide meat, milk (and cheese

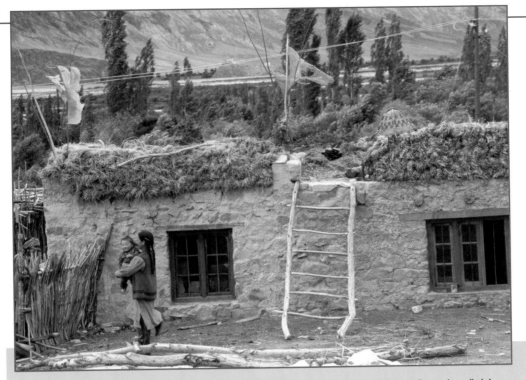

A mother and child in the Nubra Valley in the Indian Himalayas. *Nubra* means "green.," and the valley is also called the valley of flowers. The valley has been well cultivated and fertile for hundreds of years. The road to the Nubra Valley goes through the highest drivable pass in the world at Khardung La, which is about 3 miles (5 km) high.

and butter), wool, and leather for boats and clothes, dung for fuel, and a great way for carrying stuff up mountains. The Sherpa and Tibetan peoples are different in other ways, but they share these parts of their cultures.

The peoples of the Himalayas do not have the obvious high-altitude adaptations that the Andean people have. Many years ago, scientist Charles Houston said that their ability to climb was based on "willpower, motivation, and spirit." And they are highly motivated. As mountain guides they are paid well (by local standards) and do a job that brings them honor as well as danger. This has not, however, kept Sherpas from dying on the mountains of all the same things that lowlanders die of. As with the Andeans, they are just able to endure more extreme conditions than lowlanders before they have trouble.

Scientists (including Charles Houston) now know that Sherpas and Tibetans have physical adaptations for living at extreme altitudes, but it is not clear what those adaptations are or why they are different than the Andean ones. Is it because these Eastern peoples have had thousands of years longer to adapt? Or perhaps it is because all living things— plants, animals, and humans—on different continents evolve in different ways?

The Himalayan people don't have more red blood cells, but above 16,000 feet (4,875 m) they have more of the protein in the red blood cell that carries oxygen. They seem to breathe differently, inhaling more air each minute than lowlanders or Andean peoples. But they do not seem to have more oxygen in their blood, and that is what confuses scientists.

Yet scientists do know that Sherpa and Tibetan adaptations are not just acclimatization or good attitude, because of something they are able to test: the size of newborn babies. Lowlanders who move to high altitudes have much smaller babies than they would have at sea level. This is because the baby does not get enough oxygen while in its mother's womb. Andean babies, on the other hand, are only slightly smaller than babies born at sea level, because the blood traveling to the Andean baby has more oxygen in it. Tibetan mothers have babies that are almost as big as they would be at sea level, but not because they give the unborn child's blood extra oxygen. Instead they deliver more blood, faster, to the baby. They have a different adaptation from the Andean women, and it is one that works better.

Stay tuned. Modern science is still looking for more researchers who do not get sick at extreme altitudes, which is where some of these studies have to take place.

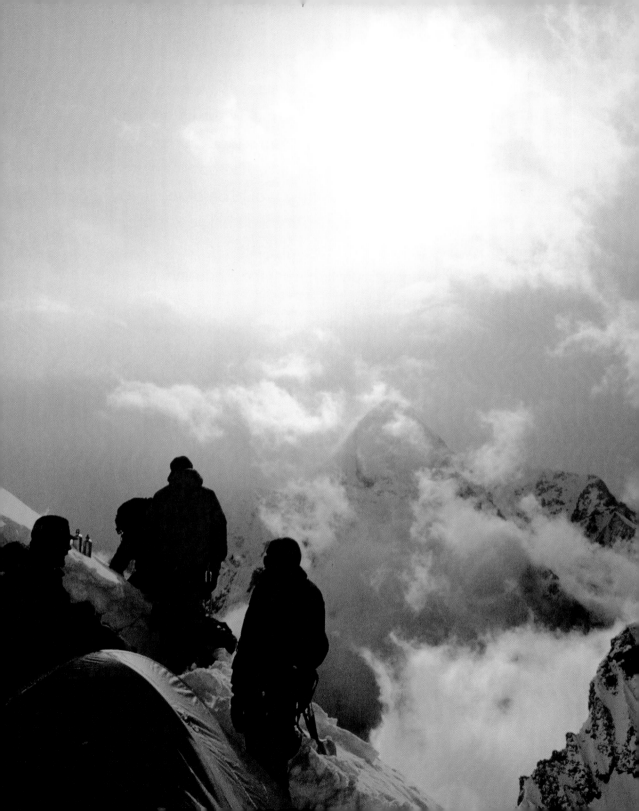

CHAPTER FOUR

ADVENTURES IN THE DEATH ZONE

When people fly from sea level to 8,000 feet (2,400 m), they may suffer from acute altitude sickness. At a high-altitude ski resort, some newly arrived vacationers may be fine, while others have headaches and a few may need a trip to the emergency room to inhale pure oxygen. If you are heading to a ski resort or mountain lodge, eat lightly and drink extra fluids when you get there. Breathe slowly and deeply. Wait a day before you ski the high peaks. Adults should not drink alcohol, as it may leave them feeling dizzy. Some aerobic exercise ahead of time may help you acclimatize, since it helps your heart pump well.

The death zone starts at 8,000 meters, which is more than 26,000 feet (although some people put it at 25,000 feet), a height that exists only in the Himalayas. However, people can certainly get themselves into trouble at lower altitudes. Many mountaineering victories or defeats take place on sheer stone cliffs in unexpected storms at much lower altitudes. But if you want extreme, the death zone is it. At 25,000 to 26,000 feet (about 7,620 to 7,925 m) the human body—no matter how well prepared—is breaking down.

CONQUERING MOUNT EVEREST

There are fourteen mountains higher than 8,000 meters. Everest is the tallest and most famous. Many people have died trying to climb Everest or have been forced to turn back. Eric Shipton, one of the best mountaineers of the 1930s, said he believed Everest would someday be climbed, but he didn't know how. Above 25,000 feet (7,620 m), mountaineering seemed impossible, even with compressed oxygen in tanks—a new invention then.

Mount Everest on a rare clear day. Half of Mount Everest is located in Nepal and half is in Tibet. Everest was named for Sir George Everest, the British surveyor-general of India at the time. The Tibetan name for Everest is Chomolungma, which is the name of the mother goddess of the earth. The Nepalese call the mountain Sargarmatha.

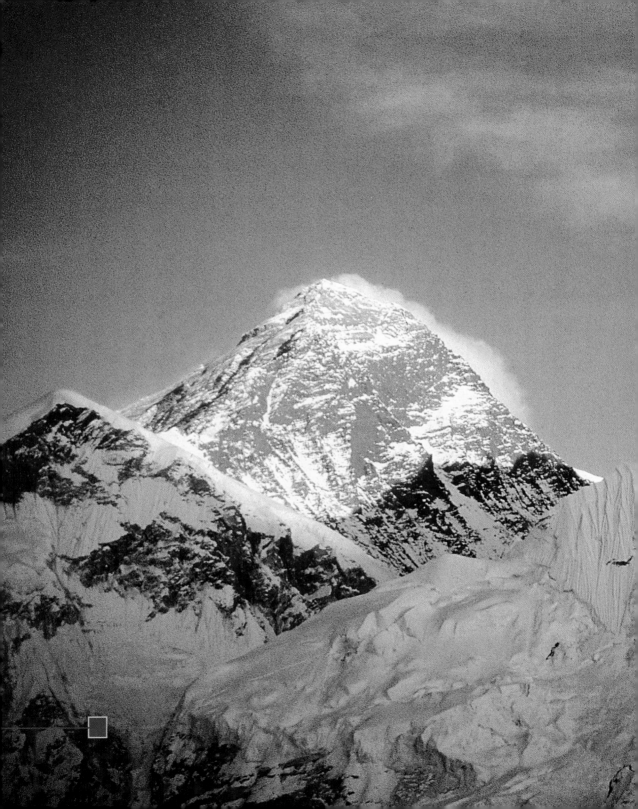

Sir Edmund Hillary, a New Zealander, and Tenzing Norgay, a Sherpa, were the first people ever to climb Everest. Part of a huge British-run expedition, they reached the top in May 1953 and became international heroes. People who remember their climb say it was as exciting as the first time people walked on the moon. Hillary and Norgay's climb was planned like a military expedition. They spoke of "conquering" the mountain, and they had hundreds of hired porters to help them, setting up camps at different altitudes and taking care of them.

Since then, some Everest climbers have climbed alone or in small groups without help. Some have climbed without oxygen tanks. But the basic plan of Hillary and Norgay's climb is used by many of the groups that climb Everest every year. There are many "paid expeditions" for which experienced climbers provide tents and equipment and

EXTREME SPAGHETTI: COOKING AT HIGH ALTITUDES

The higher you climb, the longer it takes to boil anything. Why? At sea level, water boils at 212°F (100°C). As the air becomes thinner, it presses down less on the water. This means that the water boils at lower and lower temperatures and the food cooks more and more slowly. At 20,000 feet (7,000 m) above sea level, water boils at 176°F (80°C). Instead of taking 10 minutes to cook, spaghetti will take 130 minutes.

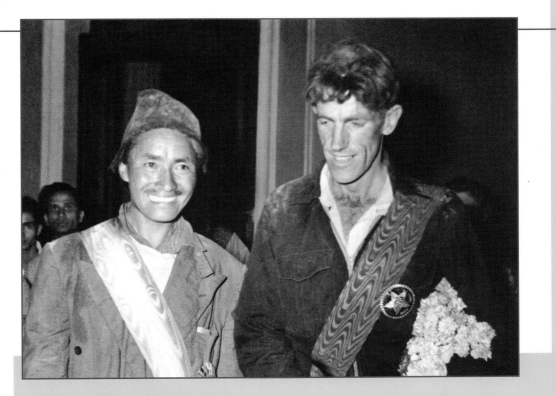

Tenzing Norgay *(left)* and Edmund Hillary pose for a portrait after being honored for their conquest of Everest by King Tribhuvan of Nepal in 1953. Norgay was presented with the Nepal Tara (Star of Nepal), a military honor, and Hillary was given the Gurkha Dakshin Bahu, the highest award in Nepal.

organize the porters and cooks. These expedition leaders obtain expensive permits from the Chinese or Nepalese governments. Climbing Everest is expensive—up to $65,000 in the late 1990s—when climbers do not have to carry tents or equipment up the mountain. On all of the paid expeditions, the guides work hard to help climbers reach the summit safely. People die anyway, every year, even though ladders and ropes now guide climbers up the mountain.

Preparation for the Death Zone

Mark Pfetzer, who attempted Everest for the first time when he was fifteen years old, prepared properly. He learned climbing techniques on a gym wall and on small cliffs. He climbed other mountains, he took courses in mountain rescue and first aid, and he spent a month at a National Outdoor Leadership School learning survival skills. He trained hard for his climbs. Living in a flat part of New England, he ran the stairs in the tallest building in his town with weights strapped to his ankles. He ran 5 to 6 miles (13 to 15.5 km) most days. He did 500 sit-ups a day and hours of other exercises. He was as big as a grown man and stronger and better prepared than most. The first time he went up Everest, he broke a rib coughing—not falling—and could barely make it down.

Pfetzer says he had always imagined that the hardest part of going up Everest would be the climbing—but for him, it was the conditions and equipment. By the time they reach the top of Everest, modern climbers are wearing long underwear and heavy socks, a one-piece down suit, gloves, over-mittens (attached to their sleeves with "keeper cords" so they can take their mittens off to tie a knot and not drop the mittens off a glacier), inner boots, boots, overboots, possibly battery-powered boot warmers, crampons (metal claws attached to boots), ski goggles, a two-way radio, six-pound (2.7-kg) oxygen tanks and an oxygen mask, and a backpack.

A few people—Pfetzer included—don't use oxygen tanks when climbing. The masks keep them from seeing well, and the tubes leading from the tank to the mask tangle them up. Also, the tanks are too small to deliver sea-level-quality air so people sometimes feel that the mask is suffocating them. Scientists say climbing without oxygen kills millions of brain cells, but climbers do not climb because it is good for them.

THE WELL-DRESSED MOUNTAINEER—1924

George Leigh Mallory and Andrew Irvine were the first Westerners to try to climb Everest and the first to die there. Mallory wore a wool jacket, sweater, and shirt, and a leather vest. His windproof overshirt was finely woven linen or cotton, which is what airplane wings were made of then. Over his pants he wore puttees—strips of fabric wrapped around his lower legs like a mummy's bandages. Over three pairs of socks, he wore leather boots with leather soles so slick he attached short nails to them. He wore goggles and carried 25-pound (11.3-kg) oxygen tanks.

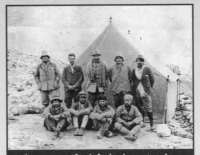

Andrew Irvine *(far left, back row)* and George Mallory *(second from left, back row)* pose with mountaineers during their 1924 Everest expedition.

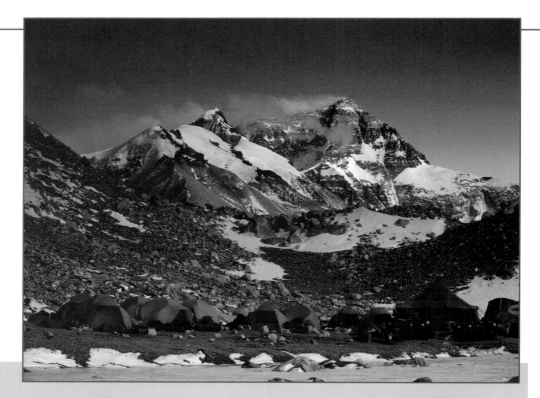

This photo shows expedition tents at the West Ridge Base Camp on Mount Everest in 1983. There are fifteen recognized routes to climb Everest, though all are dangerous. More and more climbers choose to take on Mount Everest every year, despite the fact that since 1922, over 150 climbers have died in the process.

Base Camp—and Higher

Base camp, about 17,600 feet (5,375 m) up, is where an Everest climb officially starts. Years ago, the trip to base camp could take months. Now you are brought most of the way by planes and trucks. Although the fanciest base camps now have CD players, libraries, and fax machines, base camp is not really for relaxation. The next weeks will be spent polishing climbing skills and acclimating.

People climbing Everest do not just climb up it—they go up and down like yo-yos. They rest at base camp and then climb to camp one at about 21,000 feet (9,450 m). Then they go up to camp two and stay for a few days and so on. Before they attempt the summit, they will go down to base camp or below, rest, and then go up to camp four, right below the summit, within a few days. The camps—and the climbers—are less and less comfortable as they go higher. A higher camp may consist of a tiny tent with one end pegged into rocks, while the other end sticks out over the edge.

On the guided climbs, the expedition leader may tell climbers how long to stay at each camp. They are acclimating, but they are also consuming all

HOW HIGH UP DOES THE AIR FREEZE?

The temperature drops an average of 3.5°F for every 1,000 feet above sea level. Mountain climbers can use this formula: Take the temperature at the bottom of the mountain and subtract 32°. Divide that number by 3.5 and multiply by 1,000. The answer is the number of feet above the mountain's base that the air will be freezing. (Divide the temperature by 6.5 to get freezing height in kilometers.) Therefore, if the temperature at the bottom of the mountain is 60°F (15.5°C), then 8,000 feet (2,440 m) up the mountain, the climbers need warm jackets: it's freezing up there.

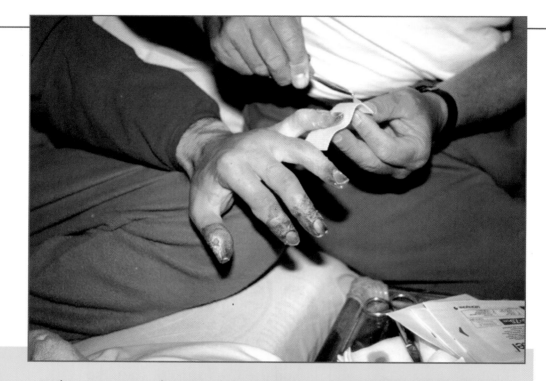

Frostbite is a common injury for mountain climbers. Frostbite develops after prolonged exposure to subfreezing temperatures or forceful winds with low temperatures. Blood vessels near the surface of the skin constrict to preserve internal body heat. This reduces the blood supply to the skin. As a result, skin tissue freezes and dies. Most frostbite occurs on the hands, face, and feet.

their body fat and many pounds of muscle. At 17,000 feet (5,200 m), a person not exercising burns more than 5,000 calories a day. Thin air makes it hard for you to digest your food. The body needs gallons of water a day to remain hydrated. At base camp, you can just about keep up with the demands the altitude is putting on your body. At higher camps you will become weaker and weaker.

As they climb, some people will also suffer high-altitude and cold-related illnesses. People who lose their goggles become snowblind—a painful blinding sunburn of the eyeball. That passes—slowly. Pulmonary edema victims blow pink bubbles when they try to breathe because their lungs have filled up with bloody fluid. In high-altitude cerebral edema, the brain fills up with fluid. Both illnesses come on very suddenly, and both are fatal unless the victim is taken to a lower altitude immediately.

People also get frostbite. Their skin and flesh—usually fingers, toes, or nose—freeze solid and later have to be amputated. Climbers often treat one another for frostbite, taking a fellow climber's frozen foot under their jackets next to their bare chest to thaw the flesh. If the foot was only beginning to freeze, this treatment is often successful.

In the death zone, the body cannot adapt. You have to urinate a lot at very high altitudes, which makes the dehydration worse, and it takes several hours to melt snow to get water. Often climbers are too tired to bother. They are also too tired to eat much. But they can't sleep. And their brains—even with oxygen tanks—are so starved for oxygen that clear thinking is impossible. Climbers feel like they are moving through molasses. They may hallucinate. And they may make deadly decisions. Mountaineers die in unexpected storms, but they also die because they are too tired to notice that they haven't fastened their equipment correctly.

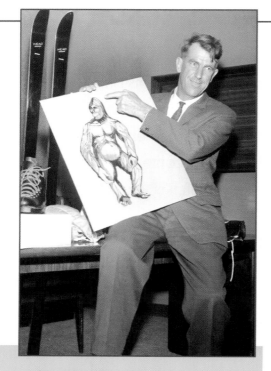

Sir Edmund Hillary in 1960, with a drawing of a hypothetical Abominable Snowman, which he hoped to capture on his next expedition. He never found one. There is no evidence that such creatures ever existed, although popular legends about them persist.

A Real Yeti?

Long before travelers saw dragons in the mountains, the ancient Greeks said the gods lived there. Moses came down from Mount Sinai with the Ten Commandments. Mountains are feared, respected, and mysterious. They are holy for many people, or hold monsters, just as outer space has Martians and E.T. and the ocean has boat-crushing creatures and beautiful mermaids.

The yeti (or Abominable Snowman) of the Himalayas is just one of the monsters who is said to live in the world's highest mountains. It is supposedly a reddish apelike creature with big feet.

Sherpas (and some Westerners) say Yetis steal people and eat whole yaks. Science cannot prove or disprove the stories for sure—some of the casts of yeti's footprints are clearly fakes, some are not.

The yeti may be a creature who is well adapted for mountain life. Or the stories of the yeti may be a human adaptation. Mountains fill people with wonder. They also kill people. When the Sherpa tell yeti stories by the campfire, they are reminding themselves what dangerous, exciting, unknown places mountains really are.

GLOSSARY

acclimatization The process by which animals (including human beings) adjust to a new environment.

adaptation The process by which living things evolve over thousands and thousands of years to fit better into their environment.

barometer A scientific instrument that measures air pressure.

conifer A cone-producing evergreen tree with needles; for instance, a pine, cedar, or spruce.

crampons A set of metal spikes attached to shoes or boots that prevents climbers from slipping on ice.

death zone The name given by mountaineers to altitudes above 25,000 to 26,000 feet (around 8,000 m), where humans can live only a short time.

deciduous Trees that lose their leaves in the autumn and grow new ones in the spring.

dehydrate To dry out; in a plant or animal, often being dried out until it is not healthy.

dormant A resting stage in which a plant or animal does not grow or move, but waits until the environment wakes it up.

frostbite The freezing of animal skin and flesh due to exposure to cold.

glacier An icy mass that forms when snow piles up for many years; the weight of the ice crushes the snow crystals until they become solid ice.

high-altitude sickness   Also called mountain sickness. The headache, dizziness, and sleeplessness that result from breathing thin air.

lichen   A crusty-looking plant without leaves, stems, or roots that can grow where other plants cannot survive.

red blood cell   The part of the blood that carries oxygen around the body.

summit   The top of the mountain; also the act of reaching the top of the mountain. "We will summit today," a mountain climber may say hopefully.

timberline/tree line   The height above sea level where trees cannot grow.

snow line   The height above sea level where snow falls all year.

ultraviolet rays   The rays from the sun (or other light sources) that can cause sunburn or skin cancer.

FOR MORE INFORMATION

The Alpine Club of Canada
P.O. Box 8040, Indian Flats Road
Canmore, AB T1W 2T8
Canada
(403) 678-3200
Web site: http://www.alpineclubofcanada.ca

American Alpine Club—National Office
710 Tenth Street, Suite 100
Golden, CO 80401
(303) 384-0110
Web site: http://www.americanalpineclub.org

The Explorers Club
46 East 70th Street
New York, NY 10021
(212) 628-8383
Web site: http://www.explorers.org

National Outdoor Leadership School
284 Lincoln Street
Lander, WY 82520-2848
(800) 710-NOLS (1-800-710-6657)
Web site: http://www.nols.edu

Parks Canada National Office
25 Eddy Street
Gatineau, Quebec K1A 0M5
Canada
(888) 773-8888
Web site: http://www.parkscanada.gc.ca

WEB SITES:

Due to the changing nature of Internet links, the Rosen Publishing Group, Inc., has developed an online list of Web sites related to the subject of this book. This site is updated regularly. Please use this link to access the list.

http://www.rosenlinks.com/lee/hial

FOR FURTHER READING

Allaby, Michael. *Biomes of the World: Mountains*. Volume 5. Danbury, CT.: Grolier Educational, 1999.

Cobb, Vicki. *This Place Is High*. New York: Walker and Company, 1989.

Krakauer, Jon. *Into Thin Air. A Personal Account of the Mount Everest Disaster*. New York: Villard, 1997.

Pfetzer, Mark, and Jack Galvin. *Within Reach: My Everest Story*. New York: Penguin Puffin, 1998.

BIBLIOGRAPHY

Andrews, Michael Alford. *The Flight of the Condor: A Wildlife Exploration of the Andes*. Boston: Little, Brown and Company, 1982

Graydon, Don, and Kurt Hanson. *Mountaineering: Freedom of the Hills*. 6th ed. Seattle: The Mountaineers, 1997.

Guterman, Lila. "The High Life: Scientists Try to Explain How the Human Body Has Adapted to Living at Extreme Altitudes,"*Chronicle of Higher Education*, August 3, 2001. Accessed July 27, 2003 (http://chronicle.com/cgi2-bin/printable.cgi).

Hare, Tony, ed. *Exploring Our World*. New York: Macmillan, 1994.

Jerome, John. *On Mountains*. New York: Harcourt Brace Jovanovich, 1978.

Klesius, Michael. "Altitude and the Death Zone," *National Geographic*, May 2003. Vol. 203:5. pp. 30–33.

Niermeyer, Susan, Stacy Zamudio, and Lorna G. Moore, "The People," in Thomas F. Hornbein and Robert B. Schoene, *High Altitude: An Exploration of Human Adaptation*. New York: Marcel Dekker, 2001.

Reid, T.R. "The Sherpas," *National Geographic*, May 2003. Vol. 203:5. pp. 42–71.

Schaller, George B. *Stones of Silence: Journeys in the Himalaya*. New York: Viking, 1980.

Sedeen, Margaret, ed. *Mountain Worlds*. Washington, DC: National Geographic Society, 1988.

West, John B. *High Life: A History of High-Altitude Physiology and Medicine*. New York: Oxford University Press, 1998.

Willis, Clint, ed. *Epic: Stories of Survival from the World's Highest Peaks*. New York: Thunder's Mouth Press, 1997.

INDEX

About the Author

Judy Levin is a children's librarian and freelance writer and editor living in New York City.

Photo Credits

Cover © Alex Steedman/Corbis; pp. 1, 3 Animals Animals © Allan, D./OSF; pp. 4–5 © David Keaton/Corbis; p. 7 Earth Scenes © Robert P. Comport; pp. 8–9 © Jim Wark/Peter Arnold, Inc.; p. 11 © Oldrich Karasek/Peter Arnold, Inc.; p. 13 © Ed Reschke/Peter Arnold, Inc.; p. 14 © Fred Bruemmer/Peter Arnold, Inc.; p. 16 © Craig Tuttle/Corbis; pp. 18–19 Animals Animals © Erwin and Peggy Bauer; p. 20 © Lior Rubin/Peter Arnold, Inc.; p. 22 © Gunter Ziesler/Peter Arnold, Inc.; p. 24 © Bill O'Connor/Peter Arnold, Inc.; p. 26 Animals Animals © Barbara Von Hoffmann; p. 27 Animals Animals © Ray Richardson; pp. 30–31 © Danny Lehman/Corbis; p. 33 © Oldrich Karasek/Peter Arnold, Inc.; p. 34 Earth Scenes © Barbara Von Hoffman; p. 35 Earth Scenes © Breck P. Kent; p. 37 © David Samuel Robbins/Corbis; pp. 40–41 © Galen Rowell/Corbis; p. 43 © Earth Scenes © Plage, D&M–Surv/OSF; pp. 45, 52 © Bettmann/Corbis; p. 47 © Hulton–Deutsch Collection/Corbis; p. 48 © Galen Rowell/ Corbis; p. 50 © Jason Burke/Eye Ubiquitous/Corbis.

Designer: Thomas Forget; Editor: Annie Sommers; Photo Researcher: Adriana Skura